Organic Body Scrubs

175 Simple Homemade Recipes For Body Exfoliation And Youthful Skin

RHODA MEYER

ISBN-13: 978-1535337878

ISBN-10: 1535337877

DEDICATION

Merry Campbell, my high school teacher; I'll never forget you!

TABLE OF CONTENTS

INTRODUCTION 1

    Exfoliation And Our Skin 1

    Body Scrubs And How To Apply Them.................... 2

    How Often Should You Exfoliate?........................... 4

    Attaining The Right Texture 5

Essential Oils.. 7

    Essential Oils & Sensitive Skin 8

Base Oils 10

Fragrance oils... 12

Butters – Shea, Cocoa, Mango 13

    The Double Boiler Method 14

SUGAR BODY SCRUBS 15

    Basic Sugar Scrub... 16

    Mango Colada... 16

    The Scent Of Christmas 17

    Grape Soufflé 17

    Simple Lemon 18

    Orange Sunrise 18

    Sweet Avocado 19

    Jasmine Rose 19

    Spicy Sugar... 20

    Chamomile Petitgrain 20

    Rosemary Lemon 21

Violet Vibrations 21

Lemon& Coconut Milk 22

Warming Gingerbread 22

Organic Citrus Sugar 23

Citrus Blast... 24

Clementine Coarse 24

Lemon Poppy Seed 25

Orange Sugar 25

Lime Margarita 26

Peppermint Sugar 26

Peppermint Citrus... 27

Rosemary Mint 27

Sugar And Spice 28

Apricot Honey Butter... 28

Peppermint Candy Cane 29

Aloe Vera 29

Lemon Milk Sugar 30

Jasmine And Aloe.. 30

Brown Sugar And Almond 31

White Chocolate &Strawberries.................................. 31

Green Tea And Honey... 32

Spring Fever 32

Sandalwood Rose 33

Wheat and Oats.. 33

Spicy Pumpkin Ginger 34

Grapefruit And Sugar... 34

Herb 35

Chocó Mocha 35

Vanilla Almond 36

Vanilla Patchouli 36

Preferred Spice Sugar 37

Soothing Brown Sugar 37

Pineapple Passions 38

Cucumber Ylang Ylang 38

Bergamot Neroli 39

Strawberry Banana Bliss 39

Tea Tree Temptations 40

Fresca 40

Snow In The Summertime 41

Maya Papaya 41

Cinnamon Celebration 42

Sweet Plum 42

Neroli Lemon Grass 43

Peach Meringue 43

Vanilla Coconut 44

Field of Flowers 44

Lavender Apricot 45

Strawberry Daiquiri 45

Sweet Sage And Lemon 46

Almond Honey 46

Lavender Lime 47

Wheat Germ 47

Lemon Poppy 48

Apple Honey 48

Vanilla Rose 49

Grapeseed And Grapes 49

Jojoba Aloe Vera 50

Bananas Forrester 50

Godiva 51

Honey Mint 51

Grapeseed And Avocado 52

Sweet Basil 52

Citrus Sandalwood 53

Almond Sugar 53

Vanilla Almond 54

Apricot Kernel 54

Nutty Sugar 55

Honey Almond Sleepy Sugar 55

Cinnamon Vanilla 56

Simple Vanilla 57

Scented Vanilla 57

Vanilla Banana 58

Vanilla Chamomile 58

Soothing Vanilla Sugar 59

Honey Sesame 59

Honey Chamomile 60

Brown Sugar Honey 60

Honey Coffee Body 61

Simple Honey Sugar 61

SUGAR SCRUBS FOR SPECIFIC BODY AREAS 62

Vanilla Sugar Lip.. 62

Peppermint Foot Sugar.. 62

Lemon Face Sugar 63

Yogurt Sugar Face Mask 63

Sugar Cookie Foot Scrub 64

Gardener's Hand Sugar Scrub... 64

CUBES AND WHIPPED SUGAR SCRUBS 65

Basic Sugar Scrub Cube 65

Simple Whipped Sugar 66

Brown Sugar Scrub Cubes 66

Vanilla Whipped Sugar 67

Whipped Shea Butter 67

Solid Shea Butter Cube 68

Whipped Super Shea Butter 69

SALT BODY SCRUBS.. 70

Chamomile Jasmine 71

Geranium 71

Artichoke 72

Mint Eucalyptus 72

Mucho Mango 73

Milk And Honey 73

Cucumber Yogurt... 74

Hazel Nut 74

Mint Salt 75

Magnesium Winter 76

Almond Milk 76

Citrus Lavender Hand Scrub 77

Lavender Mint 77

Raspberry 78

Chocolate Marshmallow 78

Summer Glow 79

Apricot 80

Cinnamon And Spice 80

Eucalyptus 81

Milk And Herbs 81

Oats And Honey 82

Watermelon Splash 82

Pomegranate 83

Totally Herbal 83

Fruit And Nut 84

Tangerine Mint 84

Ginger Lime 85

Very Berry 85

Vanilla Milk 86

Tomato Carrot 86

Cleansing Aromatic 87

Rosemary Peppermint 87

Citrus Blend 88

Tangerine 88

Egyptian Nights 89

Frankincense And Sandalwood...89

Rosemary Soy Milk 90

Pink Champagne 90

Banana Berry 91

Buttermilk..91

Autumn Harvest..92

Rose Bouquet 92

Herb Butter...93

Cucumber Lemon 93

Jasmine And Violet 94

Hot Buttered Corn 94

Autumn Harvest..95

Sweet And Salty 95

Rose Rosemary 96

Apple Pear 96

Sweet Potato 97

Cranberry Almond 97

Beer And Mayonnaise 98

Pineapple Passion 98

Egg Protein..99

Strawberry Kiwi 99

OATMEAL BODY SCRUBS 100

Simple Oatmeal 101

Grapefruit & Oatmeal..101

Baking Soda & Oatmeal 102

Almond Oatmeal Facial..102

Spicy Oat 103

Oatmeal Sunset Glow 104

Seedy Oatmeal Body Scrub.. 104

Oatmeal & Brown Sugar 105

Oatmeal And More.. 105

Oats & Coffee 106

Almonds, Avocado & Oatmeal 106

Coconut Oatmeal.. 107

Cheesy& Juicy Oatmeal 108

Oatmeal &Peels 108

Cornstarch, Oatmeal And More 109

Milky Oatmeal 109

Cucumber Oatmeal... 110

Cranberries, Coconut Super Oatmeal............................... 110

INTRODUCTION

Exfoliation And Our Skin

Our skin is a living organ. It breathes and lives and requires a lot of care—much more than any other organ in the body. It is also our body's covering. It is how other people see us. A dull and pre-maturely aged skin will make one insecure, lacking confidence and ultimately, lacking friends. On the contrary, a glowing, healthy skin makes us more youthful, vibrant and assertive.

The skin sheds up to 50,000 dead cells per minute. Not all dead cells fall off though; some of them simply build up to clog pores or leave you with a rough skin. Therefore, if you want to have a smooth and youthful skin, exfoliating is a must. In fact, the main reason for applying body scrub is for exfoliating. Exfoliating is simply the process of removing dead skin cells that clog up beneath the skin's pore in order to bring about a healthier and younger looking skin. As humans advance in age, the skin becomes rough and patchy. In exfoliation, the uneven outermost dead layer is removed to reveal a balanced smooth and fresh skin underneath.

Failure to exfoliate leaves your skin covered with dead cells that muck up the surface and gives you a dull and older look. When you repeatedly ignore this process, foundations you apply will not smooth over your skin cleanly. Moisturizers won't soak in properly as well. Facial scrub is important for breaking white -heads, cleansing the skin and dislodging build-up in the pores. It smoothens and refines the texture of the skin. It enhances blood flow to the body as well.

1

Other Exfoliation Benefits Include:

- Removal of excess oil from the skin.
- Increasing blood circulation.
- Reducing the likelihood of blackheads formation and acne breakouts.
- Reducing cellulite.
- Improving the texture of the skin.
- Minimizing wrinkles and fine lines.
- Exposing hair follicle for a closer shave.
- Allowing new cells to regenerate.
- Preparing the skin for an even tan application.
- Removing dull tanned skin.

Body Scrubs And How To Apply Them

While there are a wide range of body scrubs in the market, they contain addictives and preservatives that can damage the skin after a number of years. We need to be cautious of what we let into our skin. For many who are conscious of what they eat, it makes no sense to eat organic foods and then introduce chemicals into our bodies through our skin. This is why homemade organic body scrubs are the best! Their main ingredients are from organic substances: essential oils, base oils, fragrance oils, butters, sugars, salts, oats and many others. They do not harm the skin; rather they provide tremendous benefits to the body of which have been mentioned earlier. They are also cheaper than commercial cleansers. Homemade body scrubs is the solution to a wonderful skin and it is found in your kitchen—not the store!

The best time to apply scrubs is during a shower or a bath as the still wet skin helps the scrub to spread easily. The surface you are standing or sitting on may become slippery from the scrub's oil, so be careful!

When applying body scrubs, gently start from the feet up in an upward circular motion and then move to the legs, arms and then down your back. Finally, move up to your torso. Do not apply to sensitive areas like your pubic areas or nipples. When applying facial scrubs, be gentle and avoid your mouth and eyes. You may want to do this in front of a mirror in order not to make a mistake. Don't scrub your face too hard, this can cause damage to and hurt your skin.

Let the scrub remain on your skin for about 10 minutes to absorb its nutrients and goodness. Afterwards, rinse well with cool water. Do not wipe off the scrub so you do not end up dragging and damaging the skin. You may use a fresh wash cloth instead.

Ensure you thoroughly rinse off and that no residue scrub remains in any part of your body such as the back of your knee or the crook of your arm. Residual sugar, for instance can lead to irritation and yeast infection if it stays in the body for a while.

Gently pat yourself dry without pulling the skin. Finish up this skin pampering experience by applying a good natural moisturizer that contain alpha or beta hydroxy acids because they help in removing dead skin cells. There may be slight patches of redness after exfoliating but this will vanish once the new skin layer emerges

Exfoliating Tips

Keep These Tips At Your Fingertips:

- Wet your body in the shower from head to toe.
- Start with the soles of your feet and work your way up your body.
- Remove rough spots and calluses on your feet using a pumice stone. If you have very rough feet, add a cup of milt to a basin of

warm water, stir and soak your feet inside it for 30 minutes before entering the shower.

- Apply your scrub to your gloves or loofah. Scrub your body in a circular motion beginning with the bottoms and work your way up. Don't scrub too hard when you get to the bikini area because of the sensitive nature of the skin.
- Use a body brush to scrub your back and those places that cannot easily be reached.
- Scrub your face gently. Pay attention to your mouth and eyes but you must use an exfoliating product meant for the face because it is gentler that those made for the body.
- Remember your hands; they should look and feel soft too.
- Rinse your body using lukewarm water
- Step out of the shower
- Pat your face dry with a clean towel after exfoliating.
- Apply a moisturizing lotion all over your body

How Often Should You Exfoliate?

Most health professionals say that two times a week is sufficient. Women with oily skin need to exfoliate more frequently than women with dry skin. However, if your skin becomes irritated or dry after exfoliation, reduce the number of times you exfoliate. You may also be allergic to the products you used. Be sure to exfoliate during the winter months as the skin is more prone to the harsh drying weather conditions.

Generally, sugar scrubs works for all skin types; which is why most of the scrub recipes in this books are sugar-based. Use exfoliating cleansers that contain sugar, sea salt, walnuts, ground almonds, seeds or other grainy components.

After exfoliating, apply sunscreen if you are going out in the sun. You do not want the fresh skin to be damaged by the sun especially since it may be slightly irritated.

Body Scrubs - Dos And Don'ts

- Do not use body scrubs on sunburned, damaged or broken skin
- Do not use glass containers in the bathroom so they don't slip and break, use plastic containers instead.
- Do not allow water to get in your scrubs as it will cause the growth of mold. Store in air-tight jars in a cool, dry place.
- Discard scrubs with rancid smells or visible signs of molds.

Attaining The Right Texture

If you do not like the texture of the scrub that you have made, you can alter it to suit your preference. All you need is to just change the sugar to oil ratio and use the lighter oil to reduce the quantity of residue.

Nevertheless, the ingredients of homemade scrubs tend to separate after a while, leaving behind a slick of oil on the bathtub or shower tray when the scrub is applied. One way to overcome this issue is to add glycerine to the recipe or replace it with the oil. Glycerine helps to remove the oily residue and bind together the ingredients.

Since glycerin is a very thick and sticky liquid, it is better to replace only half of the oil with it or to rinse really well after a scrub. Additionally, keep the quantities of glycerin in any recipe low because glycerin is powerful humectants. It draws moisture into your skin from the air and has the ability to also draw out moisture from your skin.

Alternately, use a Castile soap, a vegetable- based liquid oil. It is environmentally friendly, completely biodegradable and has no chemical additives. Using a Castile soap adds an element of foaming lather for a rich scrub.

Essential Oils

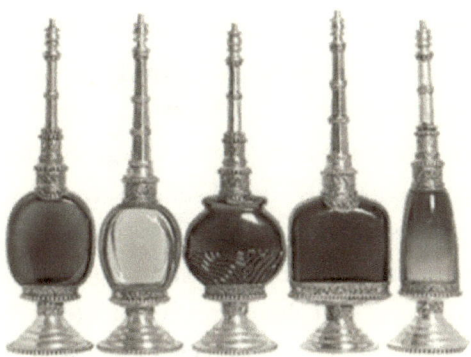

Essential oils are aromatic oils popularly used in the cosmetic industry. They are highly concentrated and have rejuvenating and healing abilities – the best treatment for your skin. These oils are extracted from the leaves, flowers, stem, seeds and roots of plants, the bark of trees as well as the peel of citrus fruits. They do not dissolve in Aloe Vera juice or water but dissolve only a little in vinegar.

If wrongly used, essential oils are harmful and this is the reason they must be kept out of children's reach. They are flammable as well and should never be placed near fires.

Essential oil should be stored in a dry and cool place. This enables it to retain its potency for 5 to 10 years. The citrus oil are an exception, however, because it only retains its healing properties for 6 to 12 months.

Be familiar with the properties and contraindications of every essential oil before using it.

Safety tips to remember when preparing your own body scrubs

- Undiluted essential oils must never be directly applied to the skin.
- They should not be taken internally because they are highly concentrated and toxic if ingested.
- Some essential oils may cause allergic reactions and skin irritation.
- Some essential oils are not suitable for pregnant women and individuals with health conditions like asthma and epilepsy.
- Essential oils like citrus oils and bergamot may cause skin sensitivity to sunlight, even when diluted. They should not be applied on sunny or extremely hot days.
- If the oil accidentally gets into your nose or eyes while working with it, flush out the affected part immediately using unscented fatty oil like olive, soybean, almond or peanut.

Many essential oils are widely used in cosmetics. You can to create your own unique blend by mixing essential oils but do not use:

➢ Lemon and Bergamot on sensitive skin
➢ Lasmine, Chamomile, Rose and Geranium during pregnancy

Essential Oils & Sensitive Skin

If you have a sensitive skin, you will need to test the essential oil you wish to add to the scrub by carrying out a skin patch test. For those who are unsure of the type of skin they have, this test will enable you to know if you have a sensitive skin or you have an allergy to the oil.

To do a skin patch test, dilute your essential oil in carrier oil. Place 1-2 drops on the inner side of your upper arm, cover with a bandage and keep it dry for 24 hours. If the skin turns red or feels hot, then it is unsafe for your use. Apply vegetable oil to the area to dilute the essential oil. You can also wash it immediately with water and mild soap but this is less effective. You may then proceed to add a new ingredient to the mix and go through the process one more time. However, if no reaction is observed, then it should be safe to use.

If you do discover you have a sensitive skin, do not scrub too hard and too often otherwise you will end up removing healthy cells and your skin will look red and feel sore. Simply rub the particles firmly but gently in circular motions. Too much exfoliation will irritate the skin.

Some essential oils like cedarwood, lavender and sandalwood are usually better on sensitive skin. If you have a food allergy, you are likely to suffer some form of skin reaction. If you have a nut allergy, for instance, avoid any nut carrier oils. Also, if you are making several batches for friends, make sure you label the jars so they know the things to avoid.

Base Oils

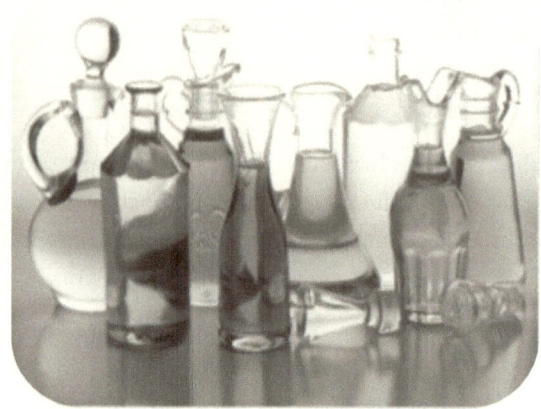

Base oils (also known as carrier oils) are primarily used in diluting essential oils before applying them to the skin as undiluted essential oils can cause burning and irritation. They are derived from fruits, vegetables, beans, seeds and nuts. They are generally cold-pressed vegetable oils without their own scent and this is why they can serve as perfect counterparts for essential oils.

Unlike essentials oils, they do not evaporate and contain little or no aroma. However, they have a shorter life span. Grapeseed, Jojoba, Sunflower, Sweet Almond, Avocado Peanut, Sesame and Apricot kernel are examples of a few of them.

Organically grown base oils which have been extracted naturally and processed minimally are the best for personal care recipes. These particular oils have not been exposed to very high temperatures, bleaching, deodorizing or chemical extraction procedures that can alter or destroy antioxidant properties, natural aromas, flavors and beneficial vitamins.

Check the labels for keywords like *cold-pressed, expeller pressed* or *refined* before you buy.Remember to always check the expiry date on the bottle and return immediately if the oil is bad. Ensure you make your purchase from reliable retailers that have a high inventory turnover.

Skin professionals sometimes use the terms slide and slip to describe the way oil product glides onto the skin. It indicates that the oil is neither rapidly absorbed nor sticky. This is the kind of base oil that is just right to use as a face or body massage oil. Soybeans oils and organic almond have thinner texture and are therefore excellent massage base oils. Jojoba oil also serves as balancing body oil.

Fragrance oils

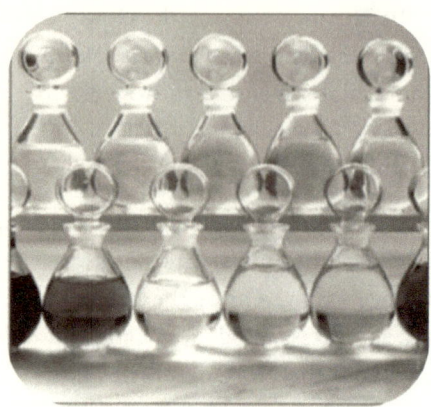

Fragrance oils, also called aroma oils, flavor oils or aromatic oils are natural essential oils that have been diluted with a carrier like mineral oil, vegetable oil or propylene glycol.

Fragrance oils are used to add a variety of scent to those fruits that do not produce essential oil such as mango, strawberry and watermelon. It is possible to even make one that will smell like chocolate! They serve as a fantastic fragrant addition to body scrubs and lotions.

However, before using these aromatics, be sure to read and follow the instructions provided on the label. And like essential oils, only a few drops are required to produce wonderful fragrant results.

Butters – Shea, Cocoa, Mango

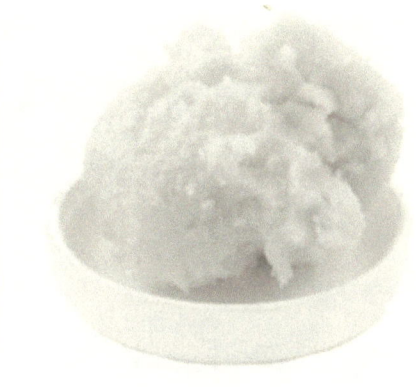

Shea nut butter is ivory-colored. It is a natural fat extraction from the fruit of the Shea tree. This fruit is called a nut and has an avocado-like seed in it. It is from this seed that Shea butter is extracted. Its uses are diverse.

- It has soothing and moisturizing effects.
- It prevents certain sun allergies.
- It protects the skin from harmful UV rays.
- It helps capillary circulation and cell regeneration.

Cocoa Butter is an aromatic solid butter from the seeds of the cacao tree which is extracted and roasted. This solid butter softens at body temperature. It adds a thick, rich and creamy consistency to body scrubs, lotions, creams and soaps which improves the skin's elasticity by helping to reduce dryness.

Mango Butter is cold pressed and rendered from the mango tree's seed kernel. It works effectively as a mild lubricant for the skin and has beneficial moisturizing properties. It is an excellent quality base ingredient perfect for body care products. It is also loaded with essential fatty acids.

The Double Boiler Method

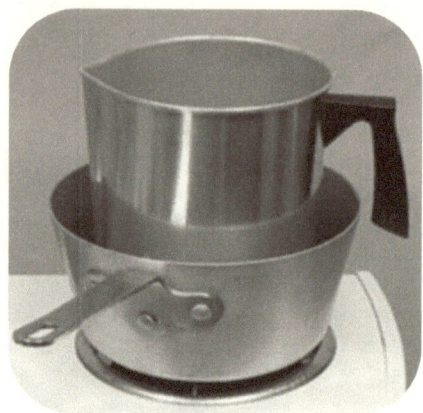

Some of the recipes in this book require the use of the double boiler method to make.

A double boiler method is effective for heating materials gently without scorching or burning them. You may either buy one but they are quite simply to make on your own.

- Get two pots, the smaller one should fit into the big one.
- Fill the big pot with some water.
- Place a one inch high sheet metal ring into the big pot. This will help the small pot to sit perfectly.
- Place the small pot on top of the big pot of water. It should not touch the water.
- As the water boils, the heat will be transferred to the smaller pot which has been filled with whatever you want to melt or cook.
- This can either be done in the oven or on the stove

SUGAR BODY SCRUBS

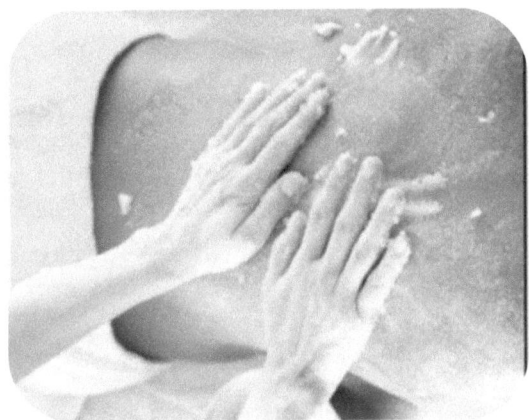

Sugar scrubs are highly recommended for individuals who have sensitive skin. They are gentler than salt and remove dead skin cells, dirt and toxin leaving the skin with a healthy and revitalized glow.

Sugar has anti-aging properties because it produces an alpha hydroxy acid known as glycolic acid which has been proven by generations to rejuvenate skin. Sugar scrubs give your skin a natural appearance and a younger glow.

Basic Sugar Scrub
Ingredients:

Organic white sugar (2 cup)

Carrier oil of choice (1 cup)

Essential oil (2-3 drops)

Directions:

Mix all ingredients well.

Transfer the now gritty paste to an air tight container using a spoon

Label, date and store in a cool place.

Shelf Life: Store in a tightly sealed container for about 3 months

Mango Colada
Ingredients:

Coconut oil (1/2 teaspoon)

Coconut fragrance oil (1/4 teaspoon)

Mango fragrance oil (1/4 teaspoon)

Pineapple fragrance oil (1/4 teaspoon)

Organic white sugar (1 cup)

Directions:

Mix oils into plastic bowl or glass

Add sugar and mix thoroughly until well blended.

Shelf Life: Store in a tightly sealed container for about a month.

The Scent Of Christmas

Ingredients:

Brown sugar (1 cup)

White sugar (1 cup)

Glycerin (½ cup)

Ground cloves (1 teaspoon)

Cocoa butter oil (½ cup)

Ground cinnamon (½ teaspoon)

Ground nutmeg (1 teaspoon)

Directions:

Combine all the ingredients in a jar, mixing well.

Label, date and store in a cool place.

Use within a couple of months.

Grape Soufflé

Ingredients:

Green grapes (1 cup)

Honey (1 teaspoon)

Egg yolk (1)

Organic white (1 cup)

Directions:

Crush green grapes to pulp. Add egg yolk and honey. Use a hand mixer to whip together

Shelf Life: Store for 24 hours in an air tight container.

Simple Lemon

Ingredients:

White sugar (2 cups)

Lemon juice(4 tablespoon)

Extra virgin olive oil (1 cup)

Vitamin E capsule

Directions:

Mix all ingredients well.

Transfer the now gritty paste to an air tight container using a spoon.

Label, date and store in a cool place.

Use scrub within 3 months.

Orange Sunrise

Ingredients:

Melted cocoa butter (2 tablespoons)

Warmed olive oil (4 tablespoons)

Orange juice (4 tablespoons)

Essential orange oil (2 drops)

Organic brown sugar (1 cup)

Directions:

Blend all the ingredients with a blender until fluffy and light.

Blend again if the mixture separates.

Shelf life: Store in a jar or a tightly-capped bottle. Refrigerate for up to 2 weeks.

Sweet Avocado

Ingredients:

Almond oil (5 drops)

Ripe avocado (1)

Organic white sugar (3/4 cup)

Directions:

Blend almond oil and pour into avocado. Add sugar and use a hand held blender to mix until smooth.

Shelf life: Use immediately.

Jasmine Rose

Ingredients:

Grape- seed oil (10 teaspoon)

Patchouli essential oil (7 drops)

Jasmine essential oil (4 drops)

Rose essential oil (2 drops)

Organic white sugar (1 cup)

Directions:

Combine all the ingredients in a bowl.

Shelf Life: Store for up to 6 months in an air tight container.

Spicy Sugar
Ingredients:

Sugar (1 cup)

Ground cloves (2 teaspoon)

Sesame oil (1 cup)

Rose essential oil (1 teaspoon)

Grated orange zest (2 teaspoon)

Directions:

Mix all ingredients well.

Transfer the now gritty paste to an air tight container using a spoon.

Label, date and store in a cool place.

Use scrub within 3 months.

Chamomile Petitgrain
Ingredients:

Chamomile essential oil (3 drops)

Petitgrain essential oil (2 drops)

Organic brown sugar (1 cup)

Dried chamomile flowers (1/4 cup)

Directions:

Combine all the ingredients in a bowl.

Shelf Life: Store for up to a month in an air tight container.

Rosemary Lemon

Ingredients:

White sugar (2 cups)

Baking soda (2 tablespoon)

Lemon juice1/4 cup ()

Extra virgin olive oil (1 cup)

Rosemary essential oil (1/8 cup)

Directions:

Combine the ingredients until mixture forms a paste-like substance.

Place in a mason jar.

Due to the olive oil ingredient, use while showering.

Violet Vibrations

Ingredients:

Coconut oil (2 ounces)

Violet fragrant oil (4 drops)

Organic white sugar (1/2 cup)

Red food coloring (optional, 1 drop)

Blue food coloring (optional, 1 drop)

Directions:

Mix ingredients together.

Shelf life: Store for up to a month in an air tight container.

Lemon& Coconut Milk

Ingredients:

Coconut oil (1/4 cup)

Coconut milk (2 tablespoon)

Sugar (1/4 cup)

Lemon zest (1 tablespoon)

1 teaspoon lemon juice (1 teaspoon)

Directions:

In a double boiler, melt the coconut oil over low heat 15- 20 seconds.

Add sugar and coconut milk, mixing until sugar is well coated.

Add lemon zest and lemon juice until all ingredients are thoroughly combined.

Store in a glass jar.

Warming Gingerbread

Ingredients:

Vegetable glycerin (1 cup)

Olive oil (1/3 cup)

Dark brown sugar (2 cups)

White sugar (1 cup)

Cocoa butter (1/3 cup)

Gingerbread fragrance oil (1 tablespoon)

Liquipar oil (5 drops)

Directions:

Combine all the ingredients in a plastic bowl, mixing well.

Transfer to wide mouth jars.

Organic Citrus Sugar
Ingredients:

Lime (1 small)

Lemon (1 small)

Coconut oil (1/2 cup)

Pure cane sugar (1 cup)

Peppermint essential oil (1 teaspoon)

Mint Leaves, lemon & lime peels (optional)

Directions:

Mix together the oil and moist ingredients.

Add the sugar. If using, add the lime and lemon peels as a garnish.

Stir, bottle and use within 3 months.

Citrus Blast

Ingredients:

Sugar (1 cup)

Jojoba oil (¼ cup)

Coconut oil (¼ cup)

Lemon essential oils (10 drops)

Lime essential oils (10 drops)

Orange essential oils (10 drops)

Directions:

Mix all ingredients well

Transfer the now gritty paste to an air tight container using a spoon

Label, date and store in a cool place.

Use scrub within 3 months.

Clementine Coarse

Ingredients:

Turbinado sugar(2 cups)

Glycerin (1 ½ tablespoon)

Almond oil (2 tablespoon)

Clementine's rind zest (1-2)

Clementine juice (2 tablespoon)

Directions:

Mix all ingredients well

Transfer the now gritty paste to an air tight container using a spoon

Label, date and store in a cool place.

Use scrub within 3 months.

Lemon Poppy Seed

Ingredients:

Raw sugar(2 ½ cups)

Juice of 2 lemons

Poppy seeds(1 teaspoon)

Olive oil (1 cup)

Directions:

Mix ingredients up.

Put it in a jar.

Apply to hands and say goodbye to those dry hands.

Orange Sugar

Ingredients:

Sugar (3/4 cup)

Orange essential oil (4 drops)

Melted coconut oil (1/4 cup)

Dried orange peel, coarsely grinded (1 tablespoon)

Olive oil (1/4 cup)

Directions:

Mix all ingredients together and place it in a clean container.

If mixture is too dry, add some more oil. If too oily, add a little more sugar.

Lime Margarita

Ingredients:

Lemon essential oil (2 drops)

Lime essential oil (4 drops)

Lime or lemon juice (½ teaspoon)

Virgin coconut oil (2 teaspoon)

Salt (1½ teaspoon)

White sugar (2 teaspoon)

Sweet almond oil or apricot kernel oil (10 drops)

Directions:

Combine the ingredients well. (The salt will stay nice and grainy but the sugar will mostly dissolve in the lime juice)

Apply to body.

Peppermint Sugar

Ingredients:

Sugar (2 cups)

Honey (½ cup)

Peppermint essential oil (1 teaspoon)

Almond oil (¼ cup)

Directions:

Mix all ingredients well.

Transfer the now gritty paste to an air tight container using a spoon.

Label and store.

Peppermint Citrus
For dry, itchy skin

Ingredients:

Granulated white sugar (1 cup)

Peppermint essential oil (10 drops)

Olive, avocado or apricot oil or a combination (1/4-1/3 cup)

2-4 tablespoon orange or grapefruit zest (2-4 tablespoon)

Vegetable glycerin (2 tablespoon)

Wild orange or grapefruit essential oil (10-15 drops)

Directions:

Mix together sugar, zest, oil and vegetable glycerin.

Gently add essential oils until the desired scent is reached.

Store in a glass container.

Rosemary Mint
Ingredients:

Sugar (2 cups)

Coconut oil (1 cup)

Peppermint essential oil (1 teaspoon)

Rosemary essential oil (1 teaspoon)

Directions:

Combine all the ingredients so it forms a paste.

Use a spoon to transfer mixture to an air -tight jar.

Label jar, date and store it in a cool and place.

Sugar And Spice
Ingredients:

Baking soda (1/2 cup)

Organic white sugar (2 tablespoons)

Organic ground cinnamon (1 teaspoon)

Organic ground ginger (1/2 teaspoon)

Organic ground cloves (1/4 teaspoon)

Almond oil (2 tablespoons)

Directions:

Combine the dry ingredients in a bowl. Then, add the almond oil. Mix them all together until well blended.

Shelf Life: Store for up to a month in an air tight container.

Apricot Honey Butter
Ingredients:

Kernel oil (10 oz apricot)

Cocoa butter (2 oz)

Organic brown sugar (1 cup)

Organic honey (1 tablespoon)

Directions:

Heat the cocoa butter in the double boiler top until it is melted.

Remove from heat and add the rest of the ingredients.

Beat with a wooden spoon till it is smooth and cooled.

Shelf life: Put in a glass jar, close tightly and refrigerate for 1 month.

Peppermint Candy Cane

Ingredients:

Granulated sugar (4 tablespoon plus 2 teaspoon)

Peppermint essential oil (3-4 drops)

Extra virgin olive oil (2 tablespoon)

Flax seed oil (1 teaspoon)

Directions:

Add together all of the ingredients, stirring well.

Sugar usually settles at the bottom so shake before using.

Aloe Vera

Ingredients:

Fine sugar (1 cup)

Aloe Vera gel(2 tablespoon)

Chamomile essential oil(1 teaspoon)

Calendula oil(1 cup)

Directions:

Mix all ingredients well

Transfer the now gritty paste to an air tight container using a spoon

Label, date and store in a cool place.

Lemon Milk Sugar

Ingredients:

Sugar (1 cup)

Milk (¼ cup)

Olive oil (2 tablespoon)

Lemon essential oil(4 drops)

Juice from one lemon

Directions:

Mix all ingredients well

Transfer the now gritty paste to an air tight container using a spoon

Label, date and store in a cool place.

Use immediately.

Jasmine And Aloe

Ingredients:

Apricot kernel oil (1/4 cup)

Cocoa butter (1 teaspoon)

Coconut oil (1 teaspoon)

Aloe Vera gel (1 teaspoon)

Jasmine fragrance oil (5 drops)

Organic brown sugar (1 cup)

Directions:

Combine ingredients into a bowl and mix thoroughly.

Shelf life: Store in glass jar for up to one month.

Brown Sugar And Almond

Ingredients:

Ground almonds (1 handful)

Brown sugar (2 tablespoons)

Honey (2 tablespoons)

Directions:

Squash almonds in a food processor. Add egg yolk and honey. Use a hand mixer and whip together.

Shelf Life: Store for up to 1 week in an air tight container

White Chocolate &Strawberries

Ingredients:

Brown sugar (1 cup)

Strawberry seed oil (1 oz)

Cocoa butter (2 oz)

Strawberry fragrance oil (20 drops)

Strawberry seeds (1 tablespoon)

Directions:

Melt the cocoa butter and add the strawberry oil.

Mix together all dry ingredients and stir.

Pour oil mixture over dry mixture, stirring well.

Green Tea And Honey
Ingredients:

Honey (2 tablespoons)

Green tea bag (1 organic)

White sugar (1 cup organic)

Almond oil (2 tablespoons)

Directions:

Place sugar in a medium sized mixing bowl. Tear open green tea bag and add to it. Stir to combine.

Next, add the almond oil and mix. Lastly, add 1 tablespoon of honey at a time and mix well.

Shelf life: Refrigerate and use within 1 week.

Spring Fever
Ingredients:

Frankincense essential oil (3 drops)

Lime essential oil (2 drops)

Rose essential oil (2 drops)

Organic white sugar (1 cup)

Directions:

Mix ingredients together in a large bowl.

Shelf Life: Store for up to 6 months in an air tight container.

Sandalwood Rose

Ingredients:

Rose essential oil (2 drops)

Sandalwood essential oil (5 drops)

Ylang Ylang essential oil (2 drops)

Organic brown sugar (1 cup)

Directions:

Combine ingredients in a bowl.

Shelf Life: Store for up to 6 months in an air tight container.

Wheat and Oats

Ingredients:

Organic white sugar (1/2 cup)

Olive oil (2 teaspoons)

Rolled oats (1/4)

Wheat germ (1/4)

Directions:

Mix ingredients together in a large bowl.

Shelf Life: Store for up to 1 month in an air tight container

Spicy Pumpkin Ginger
Ingredients:

Canned pumpkin (1/2 cup)

Fresh lemon juice (1 tablespoon)

Fresh ginger, grated (2 tablespoon)

Brown sugar (1/2 cup)

Extra virgin olive oil (1 tablespoon)

Ground cinnamon (1 tablespoon)

Directions:

In a medium sized bowl, combine all the ingredients and spoon into a jar.

Use on feet and refrigerate leftover for 3 to 4 days.

Grapefruit And Sugar
Ingredients:

Organic brown sugar (1/2 cup)

Sunflower oil (2 teaspoons)

Organic white sugar (1/2)

Vitamin E (1/2 teaspoon)

Grapefruit essential oil (3 drops)

Directions:

Mix ingredients together in a large bowl.

Shelf Life: Store for up to a day in an air tight container.

Herb

Ingredients:

Honey (1/4 cup)

Dry sage (1 teaspoon)

Dry thyme (1 teaspoon)

Dry rosemary (1 teaspoon)

Organic white sugar (1 cup)

Directions:

Combine ingredients and store.

Shelf Life: Store for up to a week in a sterilized glass jar.

Chocó Mocha

Ingredients:

Sugar (1 cup)

Ground coffee (1 tablespoon)

Macadamia nut oil (½ cup)

Cinnamon (1 teaspoon)

Cocoa powder (1 tablespoon)

Nutmeg (½ teaspoon)

Directions:

Combine all the ingredients so it forms a paste.

Use a spoon to transfer mixture to an air -tight jar.

Label jar, date and store it in a cool and place.

Vanilla Almond

Ingredients:

Whole almonds (1/3 cup)

Almond oil (1 tablespoon)

Vanilla fragrance oil (1/8 teaspoon)

Organic white sugar (1 cup)

Directions:

Pour almonds into a food processor or chopper. Then chop till particles are fine.

Combine with the sugar and oils.

Shelf Life: Store in a tightly sealed container. It lasts for up to 2 months.

Vanilla Patchouli

Ingredients:

Organic brown sugar (1 cup)

Vanilla fragrance oil (20 drops)

Patchouli essential oil (5 drops)

Ylang-ylang essential oil (5 drops)

Directions:

Mix ingredients together in a large bowl.

Shelf Life: Store for up to 6 months in an air tight container.

Preferred Spice Sugar

Ingredients:

Brown sugar (½ cup)

Turbinado sugar (½ cup)

Almond oil (¼ cup)

Coconut oil (¼ cup)

Pumpkin or apple pie spice (1 teaspoon)

Directions:

Combine all the ingredients so it forms a paste.

Use a spoon to transfer mixture to an air -tight jar.

Label jar, date and store it in a cool and place.

Soothing Brown Sugar

Ingredients:

Brown sugar (1 cup)

Rosewood essential oil (½ teaspoon)

Almond oil (½ cup)

Lavender essential oil (1 drop)

Directions:

Mix all the ingredients together until it is paste-like.

Transfer to an air -tight container.

Store it in a cool and place.

Pineapple Passions

Ingredients:

Ripe pineapple (1 cup)

Organic white sugar (1 cup)

Passionflower oil (3 drops)

Sunflower oil (1 tablespoon)

Directions:

Puree cucumber in blender. Then add oils to a mixing bowl of sugar. Mix thoroughly.

Shelf Life: Store for up to 1 week in an air tight container

Cucumber Ylang Ylang

Ingredients:

Ripe cucumber (1)

Organic white sugar (1 cup)

Ylang Ylang essential oil (2 drops)

Sunflower oil (1 tablespoon)

Directions:

Puree cucumber in blender. Next add oils to a mixing bowl of sugar. Mix thoroughly.

Shelf Life: Store for up to a week in an air tight container.

Bergamot Neroli

Ingredients:

Organic white sugar (2 ½ cups)

Almond oil (1/2 cup)

Shea butter (1 tablespoon)

Bergamot essential oil (2 drops)

Neroli essential oil (1 drop)

Directions:

Combine the almond oil and sugar in a large bowl and mix well. Then add the Shea butter and whip/ mix/ with a hand held blender on high speed for about 3minutes. You will have a grainy paste.

Shelf Life: Store in a tightly sealed container for up to 2 months

Strawberry Banana Bliss

Ingredients:

Banana (1 ripe)

Pineapples (1/4 cup)

Strawberries (1/4 cup)

Apricot kernel oil (2 tablespoons)

Organic white sugar (1 cup)

Directions:

Puree fruit in a blender. Mix fruit with sugar and oil.

Shelf Life: Store for up to 3 days in an air tight container.

Tea Tree Temptations

Ingredients:

Sunflower oil (8 teaspoons)

Jasmine oil (6 drops)

Tea tree oil (2 drops)

Neroli oil (2 drops)

Organic white sugar (1 cup)

Directions:

Mix ingredients together in a glass jar.

Shelf Life: Store for up to 2 months in an air tight container.

Fresca

Ingredients:

Tangerine fragrance oil (7 drops)

Lemon essential oil (4 drops)

Organic white sugar (1 cup)

Directions:

Combine ingredients in a bowl.

Shelf Life: Store for up to 6 months in an air tight container.

Snow In The Summertime
Ingredients:

Sugar (1/2 cup)

Olive oil (2 teaspoons)

Heavy whipping cream (1/4 cup)

Directions:

Mix ingredients together in a large bowl and use a hand mixer to mix till light.

Shelf Life: Store for up to a day in an air tight container.

Maya Papaya
Ingredients:

Papaya (1/2)

Lemon or lime juice (1/2 teaspoon)

Honey (1 teaspoon)

Organic white sugar (1 cup)

Directions:

Puree papaya in a blender. Next, add lemon juice to papaya and blend again. Add the honey and papaya to the sugar in mixing bowl. Mix well

Shelf Life: Store for up to a day in an air tight container.

Cinnamon Celebration

Ingredients:

Organic white sugar (1/2 cup)

Ground cinnamon (1/2 teaspoon)

Almond oil (1 tablespoon)

Organic brown sugar (1/2 cup)

Directions:

Combine sugars and cinnamon. Add oils and mix thoroughly.

Shelf Life: Store for up to a month in an air tight container.

Sweet Plum

Ingredients:

Plums (6)

Almond oil (1 teaspoon)

Organic brown sugar (1 cup)

Directions:

Puree the plums in a blender. Add almond oil and plums to sugar.

Shelf Life: Use immediately.

Neroli Lemon Grass

Ingredients:

Lemongrass oil (2 drops)

Neroli oil (2 drops)

Organic brown sugar (1/2 cup)

Directions:

Combine the ingredients in a bowl and mix thoroughly.

Shelf Life: Store for up to 6 months in an air tight container

Peach Meringue

Ingredients:

Peach (1 ripe)

Egg white (1)

Organic white sugar (1 cup)

Directions:

Purée the peach in a blender. Next, beat the egg white until stiff and then fold the peach purée into the egg white. Add the sugar and stir by hand.

Shelf life: Use immediately.

Vanilla Coconut
Ingredients:

Coconut oil (1 tablespoon)

Jojoba oil (2 tablespoons)

Vanilla fragrance oil (10 drops)

Coconut fragrance oil (10 drops)

Organic white sugar (1 cup)

Directions:

Combine the ingredients in a bowl and mix thoroughly.

Shelf Life: Store for up to 6 months in an air tight container

Field of Flowers
Ingredients:

Grapeseed oil (6-8 teaspoon)

Chamomile oil (2 drops)

Rose oil (2 drops)

Geranium oil (2 drops)

Jasmine oil (2 drops)

Organic white sugar (1 cup)

Directions:

Add oils to a mixing bowl of sugar. Mix thoroughly.

Shelf Life: Store for up to 1 week in an air tight container.

Lavender Apricot

Ingredients:

Organic white sugar (1/2 cup)

Plain yogurt (1/4 cup)

Mashed fresh apricots (1/8 cup)

Honey (1/8 cup)

Lavender essential oils (2 drops)

Directions:

Mix ingredients together in a large bowl.

Shelf Life: Store for 1 day in an air tight container.

Strawberry Daiquiri

Ingredients:

Very ripe fresh strawberries (1/2 cup)

Organic white sugar (1 cup)

Strawberry fragrance oil (2 drops)

Directions:

Puree strawberries and add fragrance oil and sugar.

Shelf Life: Store for a day in an air tight container.

Sweet Sage And Lemon

Ingredients:

Fresh sage (2 tablespoons)

Almond oil (4 tablespoons)

Lemon essential oil (2 drops)

Organic white sugar (1 cup)

Directions:

In a food processor, place sage or chop by hand until fine. Add the sugar and sage together in a mixing bowl and stir until sage is evenly distributed. Then add remaining ingredients and stir to mix.

Shelf life: Store and refrigerate for up to a week in an air tight container.

Almond Honey

Ingredients:

Crushed almonds (2 tablespoon)

Honey (1 tablespoon)

Organic brown sugar (1 cup)

Directions:

Place almonds in a food processor and chop until fine. In a mixing bowl, add almonds to remaining ingredients and stir to combine.

Shelf life: Store for up to a week in an air tight container

Lavender Lime

Ingredients:

Lime oil (3 drops)

Lavender oil (3 drops)

Organic white sugar (1 cup)

Directions:

Combine in a bowl and mix thoroughly.

Shelf Life: Store for up to 3 month in an air tight container.

Wheat Germ

Ingredients:

Cocoa butter (1/4 cup)

Organic wheat germ (1 tablespoon)

Apricot kernel oil (1 tablespoon)

Vitamin E oil (1 tablespoon)

Organic brown sugar (1/2)

Directions:

Use the double boiler method to melt the cocoa butter. Pour into a mixing bowl. Next, add remaining ingredients and stir to combine.

Shelf life: Store for up to 1 week in an air tight container.

Lemon Poppy

Ingredients:

Olive oil (1/2 cup)

Poppy seeds (1/2 cup)

Lemon essential oil (1/4 teaspoon)

 Organic white sugar (1/2 cup)

Directions:

Thoroughly mix all of the ingredients together.

Shelf Life: Store for 1 month in an air tight container

Apple Honey

Ingredients:

Apple, cored, quartered (1)

Honey (2 tablespoon)

Teaspoon sage (1/2 tablespoon)

Organic white sugar (1 cup)

Directions:

Place the apple slices into a food processor and chop. Then, add honey, sage and sugar.

Shelf life: Use immediately.

Vanilla Rose

Ingredients:

Rosewater (2 tablespoon)

Vanilla fragrance oil (10 drops)

Rose fragrance oil (4 drops)

Organic white sugar (1 cup)

Directions:

Combine ingredients and mix well.

Shelf Life: Store for up to 1 month in an air tight container.

Grapeseed And Grapes

Ingredients:

Grapeseed oil (8 teaspoon)

White grapes (1/2 cup)

Organic white sugar (1 cup)

Directions:

Puree grapes in a blender. Next, add grapeseed oil, grapes to a mixing bowl of sugar. Mix thoroughly

Shelf Life: Store for up to 3 days in an air tight container

Jojoba Aloe Vera

Ingredients:

Jojoba oil (2 tablespoons)

Cocoa butter (2 tablespoon)

Vitamin E oil (1 tablespoon)

Aloe Vera gel (2 tablespoon)

Organic white sugar (1 cup)

Directions:

Combine in a bowl and mix thoroughly.

Shelf Life:Store for up to 1 month in an air tight container.

Bananas Forrester

Ingredients:

Ripe banana (1)

Almond oil (1 tablespoon)

Organic white sugar (1/2 cup)

Organic brown sugar (1/2 cup)

Directions:

Puree banana in a blender. Then add sugars and blend till smooth. Pour into a bowl and mix in almond oil.

Shelf Life: Use immediately.

Godiva

Ingredients:

Godiva Chocolates (1 handful)

Organic white sugar (1/4 cup)

Peanut oil (2 tablespoon)

Fresh whole milk (2 tablespoon)

Directions:

Use the double boiler method to melt the chocolate. In a mixing bowl add the milk, sugar and peanut oil. Next, pour in chocolate and mix thoroughly.

Shelf Life: Store for up to 1 week in an air tight container

Honey Mint

Ingredients:

Mint (1 tablespoon)

Oil (1 tablespoon)

Honey (1 tablespoon)

Organic white sugar (1 cup)

Directions:

Finely chop the mint by hand or in a food processor. Add mint to sugars and other ingredients.

Shelf Life: Store for up to 1 month in an air tight container

Grapeseed And Avocado

Ingredients:

Grapeseed oil (8 teaspoon)

Avocado (1 ripe)

Organic white sugar (1 cup)

Directions:

Puree avocado in a blender. Then add grapeseed oil to a mixing bowl of sugar.

Mix thoroughly.

Shelf Life: Store for up to 3 days in an air tight container

Sweet Basil

Ingredients:

Basil oil (1 drop)

Fresh basil (2 tablespoons)

Organic white sugar (1 cup)

Directions:

Finely chop basil in food processor. Put all ingredients and mix well.

Shelf Life: Store for one day in an air tight container.

Citrus Sandalwood

Ingredients:

Safflower oil (10 teaspoon)

Orange blossom oil (5 drops)

Sandalwood oil (2 drops)

Organic brown sugar (1 cup)

Directions:

Mix ingredients together and pour into glass jars.

Shelf Life: Store for up to 3 months in an air tight container

Almond Sugar

Ingredients:

Turbinado sugar (1 cup)

Sugar (1 cup)

Vitamin E (1 teaspoon)

Almond oil (1 cup)

Directions:

Combine all of these ingredients thoroughly until it forms a paste.

Transfer to a container.

Label the container and store it in a cool and dark place.

Shelf life: 2-3 months.

Vanilla Almond

Ingredients:

Brown sugar (3 parts)

Sweet almond oil (2 parts)

Oats (1 cup)

Almond extract (1 teaspoon)

Handful of almonds ()

Essential oil of choice (2-3 drops)

Directions:

Mix all the ingredients in a food processor.

Apply to body.

Apricot Kernel

Ingredients:

Ground apricot kernel (1.5 oz)

Orange blossom floral water or citrus blend (2 oz)

Aloe Vera gel (1 oz)

Melt & pour glycerin soap (1 oz)

Sandalwood essential oil (1 drop)

Orange essential oil (2 drop)

Rice bran oil (1 oz)

Safflower oil

Directions:

Melt the soap in a double boiler. Add the safflower oil and aloe Vera gel.

Remove from heat; add the floral water and essential oils, mixing thoroughly. Add ground apricot kernel and stir frequently.

Let the mixture cool. Scrape the scrub into containers and seal for 1-2 days for ingredients to blend. Apply.

Nutty Sugar

Ingredients:

Sugar (1 cup)

Ground oatmeal (½ cup)

Macadamia nut oil (½ cup)

Ground almonds (½ cup)

Almond oil (½ cup)

Neroli essential oil (1 teaspoon)

Directions:

Mix all ingredients well.

Transfer the now gritty paste to an air tight container using a spoon

Label, date and store in a cool place.

Use scrub within 3 months.

Honey Almond Sleepy Sugar

Ingredients:

White sugar (3 parts)

Honey (1 part)

Tea (2 tablespoon)

Almond extract (1 teaspoon)

Directions

Mix all ingredients well. Ensure that it is not lumpy or break apart.

Transfer to a jar and use.

Cinnamon Vanilla
Ingredients:

Raw sugar (1/2-3/4 cup)

Brown sugar (1 cup)

Raw honey (2 tablespoon)

Sea salt (1/2 cup)

Coconut oil (1/4 cup)

Avocado oil (1/2 cup)

Cinnamon (1 teaspoon)

Vanilla extract (1-2 teaspoon)

Freshly grated nutmeg (1 teaspoon, optional)

Nutmeg essential oil (5 drops)

Cinnamon essential oil (5 drops)

Directions:

Combine the salt and sugars.

Add avocado oil, vanilla extract, essential oils and spice(s).

Add to 2 half pint jars and enjoy!

Simple Vanilla

Ingredients:

Brown sugar (½ cup)

White sugar (½ cup)

Vanilla essential oil (1 teaspoon)

grape seed oil(½ cup)

Directions:

Mix all ingredients well.

Transfer the now gritty paste to an air tight container using a spoon.

Label, date and store in a cool place.

Use immediately.

Scented Vanilla

Ingredients:

Sugar (1 cup)

grape seed oil()

Salt (½ cup)

Lemon or mint essential oils (1 tablespoon)

Directions:

Combine all of these ingredients well.

Transfer the now gritty paste to an air tight container using a spoon.

Label and store.

Vanilla Banana
Ingredients:

Sugar (1 cup)

Ripe banana mashed (1)

Vanilla essential oil (1 teaspoon)

Jojoba oil (¼ cup)

Directions:

Mash the banana lightly using a fork.

Combine with ingredients until it forms a thick paste.

Use immediately.

Vanilla Chamomile
Ingredients:

Sugar (1 cup)

Honey (¼ cup)

Jojoba oil (½ cup)

Chamomile essential oil (1 teaspoon)

Vanilla essential oil (1 teaspoon)

Directions:

Mix all ingredients well.

Transfer the now gritty paste to an air tight container using a spoon.

Label and store.

Soothing Vanilla Sugar

Ingredients:

Fine sugar (1 cup)

Honey (1 tablespoon)

Almond oil (½ cup)

Vanilla (½ teaspoon)

Vitamin E (1 teaspoon)

Directions:

Combine all the ingredients so it forms a paste.

Use a spoon to transfer mixture to an air-tight jar.

Label jar, date and store it in a cool and place.

Honey Sesame

Ingredients:

Sugar (2 cup)

Honey (1 tablespoon)

Sesame oil (1 cup)

Lemon juice (½ tablespoon)

Directions:

Mix all ingredients well.

Transfer the now gritty paste to an air tight container using a spoon.

Label and store.

Honey Chamomile

Ingredients:

Sugar (1 cup)

Chamomile essential oil (2 tablespoon)

Honey (½ cup)

Directions:

Mix all ingredients well.

Transfer the now gritty paste to an air tight container using a spoon

Label, date and store in a cool place.

Use scrub within 3 months.

Brown Sugar Honey

Ingredients:

Raw honey (1 tablespoon)

Brown sugar (1 tablespoon)

Directions:

1. In a small bowl, place the honey and brown sugar and mix well.

2. Store in a container with an air tight lid.

3. Wash face and apply about ½ teaspoon to wet skin.

4. Gently massage in a circular motion. Keep away from eye area.

5. Rinse face and pat dry.

Honey Coffee Body

Ingredients:

Very finely ground coffee (1/2 cup)

Honey (3 tablespoon)

Brown sugar (1/4 cup)

Vanilla extract (1 tablespoon)

Olive oil (2 tablespoon)

Directions:

1. Combine ingredients well.

2. Store for up to 1 month in an airtight container.

Simple Honey Sugar

Ingredients:

Sugar (1 cup)

Pure honey (1 teaspoon)

Jojoba oil (¼ cup)

ylang ylang essential oil(½ teaspoon)

Orange essential oil (½ teaspoon)

Directions:

Mix all ingredients well.

Transfer the now gritty paste to an air tight container using a spoon.

Label and store.

SUGAR SCRUBS FOR SPECIFIC BODY AREAS

Vanilla Sugar Lip
Ingredients:

Fine sugar (1 tablespoon)

Drop vanilla essential oil

Jojoba oil (1 teaspoon)

Directions:

Mix all ingredients well

Transfer the now gritty paste to an air tight container using a spoon

Label, date and store in a cool place.

Peppermint Foot Sugar
Ingredients:

Sugar (1 cup)

Peppermint essential oil (1 teaspoon)

Jojoba oil (½ cup)

Directions:

Mix all ingredients really well until mixture forms a paste.

Spoon into a glass container with a lid that seals.

Use the scrub within a couple of months.

Lemon Face Sugar
Ingredients:

Fine sugar (½ cup)

Juice of lemon (½)

Honey (1 tablespoon)

Evening primrose oil (1 tablespoon)

Directions:

Combine all the ingredients so it forms a paste.

Use a spoon to transfer mixture to an air -tight jar.

Label jar, date and store it in a cool and place.

Use within 3 months.

Yogurt Sugar Face Mask
Ingredients:

Sugar (2 teaspoon)

Plain yogurt (3 teaspoon)

Directions:

Combine all the ingredients so it forms a paste.

Use a spoon to transfer mixture to an air -tight jar.

Use and discard any left. Do not store.

Sugar Cookie Foot Scrub

Ingredients:

Packed brown sugar (1/3 cup)

Granulated white sugar (2/3 cup)

Vanilla extract (1 tablespoon)

Olive oil (1/2 cup)

Directions:

Combine white sugar & brown sugar in a medium sized bowl.

Whisk together until well combined.

Add olive oil and vanilla extract and then use a fork to mash together until the oil is incorporated into the sugar mixture.

Pack the mixture into an air tight jar.

Label, date and store in a cool place.

Gardener's Hand Sugar Scrub

Ingredients:

Sugar (1 cup)

Vitamin E(½ teaspoon)

Almond oil (½ cup)

Lavender (1 teaspoon)

Directions:

Mix all ingredients really well until mixture forms a paste.

Spoon into a glass container with a lid that seals.

Use the scrub within a couple of months.

CUBES AND WHIPPED SUGAR SCRUBS

Basic Sugar Scrub Cube

Ingredients:

Sugar (2 parts)

Melt &pour soap base (1 part)

Carrier oil (1 part)

Essential oil of choice

Directions:

Cube the melt& pour soap and then put in a glass jug or bowl.

Melt the soap for 20-30 seconds in the microwave and stir.

Add essential oil, any preferred coloring, the oil and then mix.

Add the sugar, stirring quickly until fully combined. Pour into the mold quickly before it solidifies.

The mixture will take about 1 hour to set at room temperature.

Once set, just pop out cubes if an ice cube tray was used. If plastic container was used, turn out the block and then cut to the desired size and number of pieces. You can also use a melon baller to make little scrub balls.

Keep these individual portions for use or package up a lovely gift.

Simple Whipped Sugar

Ingredients:

Sugar (1 cup)

Vitamin E oil

Carrier oil (½ cup)

Water (1 tablespoon)

Essential oils

Directions:

Put the sugar, water and carrier oil in a bowl and whisk until mixture is light and fluffy.

Add essential oils, vitamin E and mix well.

Transfer to a wide mouthed jar.

Brown Sugar Scrub Cubes

Ingredients:

Brown sugar (1 cup)

Honey (1 teaspoon)

Avocado oil (½ cup)

Melted melt & pour soap (½ cup)

Essential oil (1 teaspoon)

Directions:

Mix all ingredients well.

Transfer the now gritty paste to an air tight container using a spoon

Label, date and store in a cool place.

Use scrub within 3 months.

Vanilla Whipped Sugar

Ingredients:

Sugar (1 cup)

Vanilla extract (½ teaspoon)

Jojoba oil (½ cup)

Directions:

Combine all ingredients and whisk until thick and creamy.

Whipped Shea Butter

Ingredients:

Sugar (1 cup)

Almond oil (¼ cup)

Shea butter (½ cup)

vitamin E oil(½ teaspoon)

Directions:

Put the Shea butter in the microwave to soften.

Using a mixer, whisk until thick and creamy.

Gradually add the almond oil in stages, mixing well between each addition.

Now, add vitamin E and then mix thoroughly.

Gradually add the sugar in stages, mixing until the desired consistency is attained.

Solid Shea Butter Cube

Ingredients:

Refined Shea butter (4 oz)

Shea butter soap base (2.5 oz)

Fractionated coconut oil (2 tablespoon)

White sugar (16 oz)

Essential oils of choice(½ tablespoon)

Pinch of mica (optional)

Directions:

Weigh out the melt and pour soap base then melt. Weigh out Shea butter and melt.

Add the Shea butter into the melt & pour soap base and stir. Add the fractionated coconut oil and essential oils and stir.

Pour the sugar into the soap/ Shea mixture, mixing well. Scoop into mold and use a spatula to level. Refrigerate until solidified.

Remove the scrub gently from the molds. Remove plastic wrap from scrub. Cut the scrub into cubes with a Chef's knife.

Place cubes in an airtight jar until use.

Whipped Super Shea Butter

Ingredients:

Raw Shea butter (1/2 cup)

Apricot kernel or sweet almond (1/3 cup)

Rosemary extract (1/8 teaspoon)

Corn starch to make the butter feel less greasy (1 teaspoon)

Grapefruit or rosemary essential oil (2-3 drops)

Sugar (1/2 –1 cup)

Directions:

Place Shea butter in a mixing bowl and then beat until the butter is creamy.

If butter is too hard, put in the microwave to soften for 15 seconds but don't melt.

Add the carrier oil a little at a time and blend fully between additions.

Add the rosemary extract and then the cornstarch and essential oil, blending well.

Mix in the sugar gradually until the desired consistency is achieved.

SALT BODY SCRUBS

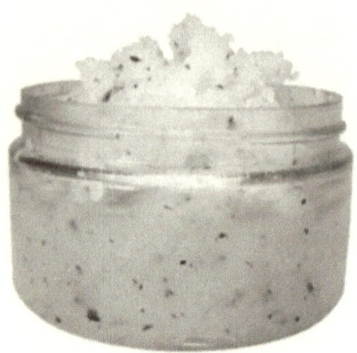

Salt scrubs enhance the circulation to the skin. They are coarser than sugar-based scrubs and have more exfoliating power.

People who have sensitive skin should NOT use salt scrubs. It is advisable to begin your exfoliating routine once a week.

Chamomile Jasmine

Ingredients:

Dried chamomile leaves (1 tablespoon)

Jasmine essential oil (1 tablespoon)

Crushed organic sea salt (1 cup)

Jojoba oil (3 tablespoon)

Directions:

Combine ingredients in mixing bowl and stir.

Shelf Life: Store for up to 1 week

Geranium

Ingredients:

Crushed organic sea salt (1/2 cup)

Geranium essential oil (4 drops)

Shea butter (2 tablespoons)

Apricot kernel oil (2 tablespoons)

Directions:

Use the double boiler method to melt Shea butter. Add to oils and sea salt

Shelf Life: Store for up to 6 months.

Artichoke

Ingredients:

Fresh artichoke hearts (1)

Canola oil (2 teaspoon)

Crushed organic sea salt (1 cup)

Fresh lemon juice (1 teaspoon)

Directions:

Mash cooked artichoke hearts in a glass bowl and mix with lemon and oil.

Stir well till smooth paste.

Shelf Life: Store for 1 week.

Mint Eucalyptus

For the feet

Ingredients:

2 cup fine or medium ground sea salt (for rougher feet, use coarser salt)

1 cup coconut oil

15 drops peppermint essential oil

25 drops eucalyptus essential oil

Directions:

1. Combine all the ingredients in a jar.

2. Apply scrub with bare hands or wash cloths.

3. Scrub feet gently until smooth and supple and then rinse.

Mucho Mango

Ingredients:

Ripe mango (1)

Mango butter (2 tablespoon)

Crushed organic sea salt (1 cup)

Apricot kernel oil (2 tablespoons)

Directions:

Use the double boiler method to melt mango butter. Puree mango in a blender.

Mix all ingredients in a bowl and stir well.

Shelf Life: Store for 2 months.

Milk And Honey

Ingredients:

Milk or cream (1/4 cup)

Crushed organic sea salt (1 cup)

Honey (1/4 cup)

Directions:

Mix honey and milk (or cream) in an enamel pan or a small glass.

Warm until the honey melts. Remove from heat.

Shelf Life: Store for 1 week.

Cucumber Yogurt

Ingredients:

Cucumber (1 tablespoon)

Parsley (1 tablespoon)

Yogurt (1 tablespoon)

Crushed organic sea salt (1cup)

Directions:

Combine ingredients in mixing bowl and stir.

Hazel Nut

Ingredients:

Crushed organic sea salt (1/2 cup)

Hazel nut oil (2 tablespoon)

Crushed hazel nuts (1/4)

Directions:

Mix all ingredients.

Shelf Life: Store for a week in an air tight container.

Mint Salt

This moisturizing scrub doubles as soap

Ingredients:

Epsom salts (3/8 cup)

Liquid castile soap (1/8 cup)

Glycerin soap base (1/2 oz)

Jojoba oil (1 tablespoon)

Sunflower (1/8 cup)

Peppermint essential oil (4 drops)

Tea tree essential oil (2 drops)

Aloe gel (1 teaspoon, optional)

Green or blue mica powder for color (optional)

Directions:

Melt the glycerin soap base.

Add oils and liquid soap. Remove from heat.

Add essential oils, salt, aloe and color. (Mix the powder with some oil before you mix it in).

Plop the now thick mixture into a plastic or glass container. Let it cool.

Magnesium Winter

Ingredients

Epsom salt (1 cup)

Almond oil or olive oil (¼ cup)

Liquid castile soap (1 teaspoon)

Peppermint and citrus essential oils (10-15 drops)

Directions

Mix all ingredients together in a small bowl.

Add essential oils until desired fragrance is achieved.

Store in an airtight jar.

Use a teaspoon sized amount to exfoliate body as needed.

Rinse after use.

Use within 3 months.

Almond Milk

Ingredients:

Almond oil (1/4 cup)

1 cup crushed organic sea salt (1 cup)

Almond milk (1/4 cup)

Directions:

Mix ingredients until well mixed.

Shelf Life: Store for 1 week.

Citrus Lavender Hand Scrub

Ingredients

Dried lavender (1 tablespoon)

Olive oil (⅓ Cup)

Lemon zest (2 teaspoon)

Kosher salt (1 cup)

Freshly squeezed lemon juice from 1 small lemon (1 tablespoon)

Directions

 In a small pan over low heat, place the lavender and olive oil to warm for about 5 minutes.

Turn heat off and allow the infused oil cool to room temperature.

Combine salt, lemon juice and lemon zest in a small bowl.

Stir in the infused oil

Transfer scrub to a glass jar with an airtight lid and then store.

Lavender Mint

Ingredients:

Dried lavender (2 tablespoons)

Mint (1 tablespoon)

Crushed organic sea salt (1cup)

Canola oil (4 tablespoons)

Directions:

Place mint on a cutting board and finely chop. Continue with salt, oil and dried lavender.

Shelf Life: Store for 3 months.

Raspberry
Ingredients:

Fresh raspberry (1/2 cup)

1 cup crushed organic sea salt (1 cup)

Sunflower oil (4 tablespoons)

Directions:

Combine ingredients in a food processor.

Shelf Life: Store in a glass jar for a week.

Chocolate Marshmallow
Good for dry skin

Ingredients:

Shea butter (4 oz.)

Cocoa butter(4 oz.)

Fractionated coconut oil(4 oz.)

Natrasorb(2 tablespoon)

Turbinado sugar(1 1/4 cup)

dendritic salt(1/4 cup)

polysorbate 20(1 teaspoon)

Milk chocolate fragrance oil(1 teaspoon)

Marshmallow root powder (1 tablespoon)

Milk powder (1 tablespoon)

Cocoa powder (1 tablespoon)

Directions:

Heat the oils and butters until melted.

Blend the additives, Natrasorb and powders in a separate bowl.

Mix the polysorbate 20 and fragrance and add to the Natrasorb.

Now add the turbinado sugar, mix well and gently pour oil over the sugar blend.

Let the mixture cool. Store and use at room temperature.

Summer Glow
Ingredients:

Crushed organic sea salt (1/2 cup)

Mango butter (2 tablespoons)

Shea butter (2 tablespoons)

Cocoa butter (2 tablespoons)

Fine silver glitter (1/2 tablespoons)

Directions:

Use the double boiler method to melt all the butters together.

Combine all ingredients in a bowl and use a hand mixer to mix well.

Shelf Life: Store for up to 2 months in an air tight container.

Apricot

Ingredients:

Crushed organic sea salt (1/2 cup)

Fresh apricot (1/2 cup)

Apricot fragrance oil (2 drops)

Directions:

Puree apricot in blender. Mix all ingredients in a bowl and stir well.

Shelf Life: Store for 1 week in an air tight container

Cinnamon And Spice

Ingredients:

Sunflower oil (4 tablespoon)

Crushed organic sea salt (1 cup)

Ground cinnamon (2 tablespoon)

Ground nutmeg (1 tablespoon)

Directions:

Combine ingredients in a bowl and mix thoroughly.

Shelf Life: Store for up to 2 months in an air tight container.

Eucalyptus

Ingredients:

Olive oil (4 tablespoon)

Crushed organic sea salt (1/2 cup)

Eucalyptus essential oil (2 drops)

Directions:

Combine ingredients in a bowl and mix thoroughly.

Shelf Life: Store for up to 6 months in an air tight container.

Milk And Herbs

Ingredients:

Olive oil (4 tablespoon)

Crushed organic sea salt (1/2cup)

Powdered goats milk (2 tablespoon)

Dried thyme (1 tablespoon)

Dried rosemary (1 tablespoon)

Directions:

Combine ingredients in a bowl and mix thoroughly.

Shelf Life: Store for 2 weeks in an air tight container.

Oats And Honey

Ingredients:

Powdered oats (1/4 cup)

Crushed organic sea salt (1/2 cup)

Honey (1/4 cup)

Sweet almond (2 tablespoons)

Directions:

Mix powdered oats and salt. Add the honey and then the oil.

Mix until fully combined.

Shelf Life: Store for 2 months in an air tight container.

Watermelon Splash

Ingredients:

Crushed organic sea salt (1/2 cup)

Fresh watermelon (1/2 cup)

Directions:

Combine ingredients in a bowl and mix well.

Shelf Life: Store for up to 1 week in an air tight container.

Pomegranate

Ingredients:

Apricot kernel oil (4 tablespoon)

Crushed organic sea salt (1 cup)

Pomegranate juice (2 tablespoon)

Pomegranate fragrance oil (3 drop)

Directions:

Combine ingredients in a bowl and mix well.

Shelf Life: Store for up to 2 weeks in an air tight container.

Totally Herbal

Ingredients

Norwegian kelp powder (1/2 cup)

bladderwrack powder (1/2 cup)

Dead Sea clay (1/3 cup)

Dead Sea salt (1/2 cup)

Walnut oil (1/2 cup)

Emu oil (1/3 cup)

Jojoba oil (1 cup)

liquipar oil (10 drops)

T-50 vitamin E oil (1 tablespoon)

Directions:

Combine ingredients in a large bowl and then mix thoroughly.

If mixture is too wet, add more clay and if too dry, add more emu oil until it is a little slushy.

Fruit And Nut

Ingredients:

Crushed almonds (1/2 cup)

Crushed organic sea salt (1/2 cup)

Raisons (2 tablespoons)

Dried cranberries (2)

Almond oil (2 tablespoon)

Directions:

Combine ingredients in a bowl and mix thoroughly.

Shelf Life: Store for 2 months in an air tight container.

Tangerine Mint

Ingredients:

Olive oil (4 tablespoon)

Cup crushed organic sea salt (1/2cup)

Tangerine fragrance oil (2 drops)

Spearmint essential oil (2 drops)

Directions:

Combine all ingredients and mix well.

Shelf Life: Store for up to 6 months in an air tight container.

Ginger Lime
Ingredients:

Crushed organic sea salt (1 cup)

Ground ginger (1 teaspoon)

Fresh lime juice (1 teaspoon)

Macadamia nut oil (4 tablespoon)

Directions:

Combine all ingredients and mix well.

Shelf Life: Store for up to 2 weeks in an air tight container.

Very Berry
Ingredients:

Strawberry fragrance oil (2 drops)

Crushed organic sea salt (1 cup)

Raspberry fragrance oil (2 drops)

Sweet almond oil (2 tablespoon)

Vitamin E oil (2 tablespoon)

Directions:

Combine all the ingredients in a bowl and stir well.

Shelf Life: Store for up to 3 months in a glass jar.

Vanilla Milk

Ingredients:

Vanilla extract (2 tablespoon)

Crushed organic sea salt (1 cup)

Milk (4 tablespoons)

Powdered goat's milk (2 tablespoon)

Directions:

Mix all the ingredients in a glass bowl.

Shelf Life: Store for up to 1 week in a glass jar.

Tomato Carrot

Ingredients:

Crushed organic sea salt (1/2 cup)

Ripe tomato (1)

Carrot juice (1/4)

Directions:

Puree carrot juice and tomato. Add salt and beat with a hand mixer.

Shelf Life: Store for up to 1 week in an air tight container.

Cleansing Aromatic

Ingredients:

Epsom salts (1/4 cup)

Sea salt (1/4 cup)

Borax (1 tablespoon)

Almond oil (1/4 cup)

Baking soda (1 tablespoon)

Geranium essential oil (8 drops)

Lavender essential oil (4 drops)

Directions:

Mix salts in canning jar. Add borax and baking soda and mix again.

Add the essential oils to almond oil then mix with salts mixture.

Add the oils to the mixture and then mix well and store.

Rosemary Peppermint

Ingredients:

Dried rosemary (2 tablespoon)

Crushed organic sea salt (1 cup)

Peppermint fragrance oil (3 drops)

Directions:

Combine all ingredients in a mixing bowl.

Shelf Life: Store for 6 months.

Citrus Blend

Ingredients:

Mango butter (2 tablespoon)

Crushed organic sea salt (1 cup)

Orange essential oil (2 drops)

Lemon essential oil (2 drops)

Grapefruit essential oil (2 drops)

Almond oil (2 tablespoon)

Directions:

Use a double boiler to melt mango butter and add to the other ingredients.

Shelf Life: Store for up to 6 months in an air tight container.

Tangerine

Ingredients:

Tangerine essential oil (2 drop)

Crushed organic sea salt (1 cup)

Dried orange peel powder (4 tablespoons)

Apricot kernel (2 tablespoons)

Directions:

Mix all the ingredients and stir well.

Shelf Life: Store for up to 3 months in a glass jar.

Egyptian Nights

Ingredients:

Crushed organic sea salt (1/2 cup)

Egyptian musk fragrance oil (3 drops)

Epsom salt (1/4 cup)

Directions:

Combine all ingredients and mix well

Shelf Life: Store for up to 6 months in an air tight container.

Frankincense And Sandalwood

Ingredients:

Frankincense essential oil (2 drops)

Crushed organic sea salt (1 cup)

Sandalwood essential oil (2 drops)

Vegetable oil (2 tablespoon)

Directions:

Mix all ingredients in a bowl and stir well.

Shelf Life: Store for up to 3 months in a glass jar.

Rosemary Soy Milk
Ingredients:

Soy milk (2 tablespoon)

Crushed organic sea salt (1 cup)

Dried rosemary (4 tablespoons)

Canola oil (4 tablespoons)

Directions:

Mix all ingredients in a glass bowl.

Shelf Life: Store for up to 1 week in a glass jar.

Pink Champagne
Ingredients:

French pink champagne (2 tablespoon)

Crushed organic sea salt (1 cup)

Epsom salt (2 tablespoon)

Directions:

Mix all ingredients in a glass bowl.

Shelf Life: Store for up to 2 weeks in a glass jar.

Banana Berry

Ingredients:

Ripe banana (1)

Strawberry fragrance oil (3 drops)

Crushed organic sea salt (1/2 cup)

Fresh strawberries (1/4)

Directions:

Combine all ingredients and mix with a hand mixer.

Shelf Life: Store for 2 days in an air tight container

Buttermilk

Ingredients:

Crushed organic sea salt (1/2 cup)

Lemon tea tree essential oil (1 teaspoon)

Buttermilk (2 teaspoon)

Yogurt (2 teaspoons)

Directions:

Mix all ingredients in a mixing bowl.

Shelf Life: Store for a week in an air tight container.

Autumn Harvest

Ingredients:

Peach fragrance oil (3 drops)

Bergamot Essential Oil (3 drops)

Vanilla Essential Oil (3 drops)

Range fragrance oil (3 drops)

Crushed organic sea salt (1/2 cup)

Directions:

Combine all ingredients and mix.

Shelf Life: Store for up to 6 months in an air tight container.

Rose Bouquet

Ingredients:

Pink Rose Petal Powder (2 tablespoon)

Crushed organic sea salt (1 cup)

Rose fragrance oil (3 drops)

Rosewater Powder (1 tablespoon)

Directions:

Combine all ingredients in a mixing bowl.

Shelf Life: Store for 2 months.

Herb Butter

Ingredients:

Dried mint (2 teaspoon)

Dried sage (2 teaspoon)

Dried rosemary (2 teaspoon)

Cocoa butter (6 ounces)

Crushed organic sea salt (1 cup)

Directions:

Combine all ingredients in a mixing bowl.

Shelf Life: Store for 6 months.

Cucumber Lemon

Ingredients:

Crushed organic sea salt (1/2 cup)

Ripe cucumber (1)

Fresh squeezed lemon juice (2 tablespoon)

Yogurt (2 tablespoon)

Lemon essential oil (2 drops)

Directions:

Chop cucumber into small pieces, add yogurt and lemon then blend to make a paste.

Next, remove from food processor and add salt. Mix thoroughly.

Shelf Life: Store for a week in an air tight container.

Jasmine And Violet

Ingredients:

Jasmine essential Oil (3 drops)

Violet essential Oil (3 drops)

Crushed organic sea salt (1/2 cup)

Directions:

Combine ingredients in a bowl and mix.

Shelf Life: Store in an air tight container for 6 months.

Hot Buttered Corn

Ingredients:

Crushed organic sea salt (1/2 cup)

Butter (1 teaspoon)

Canola oil (1 teaspoon)

Corn meal (11/4 cup)

Water (11/4 cup)

Directions:

Microwave the cornmeal and water for 1 minute on high temperature.

Combine the remaining ingredients in a mixing bowl.

Leave to cool till room temperature.

Shelf Life: Store in an air tight container for a month.

Autumn Harvest

Ingredients:

Peach fragrance oil (3 drops)

Bergamot Essential Oil (3 drops)

Vanilla Essential Oil (7drops)

Orange fragrance oil (3 drops)

Crushed organic sea salt (1/2 cup)

Directions:

Combine ingredients in a bowl and mix.

Shelf Life: Store for up to 6 months in an air tight container.

Sweet And Salty

Ingredients:

Crushed organic sea salt (1/2 cup)

Organic white sugar (1/2 cup)

Directions:

Combine all ingredients and beat.

Shelf Life: Store for up to 1 week in an air tight container.

Rose Rosemary

Ingredients:

Rose essential oil (3 drops)

Crushed organic sea salt (1/2 cup)

Dried rosemary (2 tablespoon)

Directions:

Combine ingredients and beat with a hand mixer.

Shelf Life: Store in an air tight container for a week.

Apple Pear

Ingredients:

Crushed organic sea salt (1/2 cup)

Small fresh green apple (1)

Small pear (1)

Fresh lemon (2 teaspoons)

Apple fragrance oil (2 drops)

Pear fragrance oil (2 drops)

Directions:

Puree fruit with lemon juice in a blender. Then, combine all ingredients and mix thoroughly.

Shelf Life: Store for a day in an air tight container.

Sweet Potato

Ingredients:

Crushed organic sea salt (1/2 cup)

Cooked sweet potato (1/2 cup)

Ground cinnamon (1 teaspoon)

Directions:

Combine ingredients and beat with a hand mixer.

Shelf Life: Store in an air tight container for to 2 weeks.

Cranberry Almond

Ingredients:

Crushed almonds (1/2 cup)

Crushed organic sea salt (1/2 cup)

Cranberries (2)

Almond oil (2 tablespoon)

Directions:

Combine ingredients in a bowl and mix well.

Shelf Life: Store in an air tight container for 2 months.

Beer And Mayonnaise

Ingredients:

Beer (1/2 cup)

Crushed organic sea salt (1/2 cup)

Mayonnaise (2 tablespoon)

Directions:

Combine all ingredients and beat with a hand mixer.

Shelf Life: Store in an air tight container for 2 weeks.

Pineapple Passion

Ingredients:

Pineapple fragrance oil (3 drops)

Passion fruit fragrance oil (3 drops)

Crushed organic sea salt (1/2 cup)

Fresh pineapple (1/2 cup)

Directions:

Puree fruits in the blender. Mix all ingredients in a bowl and beat with a hand mixer.

Shelf Life: Store in an air tight container for a week.

Egg Protein

Ingredients:

Crushed organic sea salt (1/2 cup)

Large egg (1)

Protein powder (2 tablespoon)

Directions:

Combine ingredients and beat with a hand mixer.

Shelf Life: Store in an air tight container for 2 months.

Strawberry Kiwi

Ingredients:

Strawberry fragrance (3 drops)

Crushed organic sea salt (1/2 cup)

Fresh strawberries (1/4 cup)

Ripe kiwi (1)

Directions:

Combine ingredients and beat with a hand mixer.

Shelf Life: Store for up to 1 week in an air tight container.

OATMEAL BODY SCRUBS

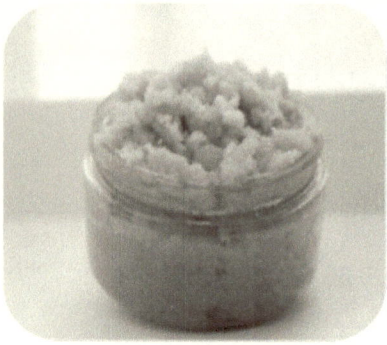

Oats contain grainy substances which have been proven to be very good for facial scrubs. Oats also absorb and remove surface dirt and skin impurities.

Using scrubs made with this wonderful ingredient will help in treating several skin conditions. It works well for dry and itchy skin and is just right for sensitive skin. Scrubs used with oatmeal will leave your skin soft, silky smooth and hydrated.

Before applying any oatmeal scrub, it is advisable to wash your face with lukewarm water. The scrub can also be used immediately after a shower. This opens up the pores and prepares the skin for improved result.

Simple Oatmeal

Ingredients:

Oatmeal (1 tablespoon)

Warm water or more (3 tablespoon)

Directions:

Combine ingredients.

Wait for about 10 minutes until oats soften and then use.

Grapefruit & Oatmeal

The use of citrus with oatmeal is a wonderful combination that helps in stimulating, toning and exfoliating the skin.

Ingredients:

Fresh Grapefruit (1)

Oatmeal (2 tablespoons)

Directions:

Squeeze juice and pulp out of grapefruit.

Mix with oatmeal till it forms a smooth paste.

Baking Soda & Oatmeal

The baking soda in this oatmeal scrub serves as a booster. It will soothe your skin in a pleasantly surprising way.

Ingredients

Oatmeal (2 heaping tablespoons)

Baking soda (1 teaspoon)

Directions:

Mix ingredients and add sufficient water to make a sticky paste.

Scrub your face in circular motions, massaging it gently to your skin. Rinse off with lukewarm water.

Almond Oatmeal Facial

Ingredients

Almonds (1/4 cup)

1/4 cup oatmeal (1/4 cup)

Cornstarch (1 tablespoon)

chamomile flower tea (1 tablespoon, optional)

Directions

Add all the ingredients to a blender or food processor and process until the mixture looks like a fine mealy-textured powder.

Transfer to small glass jars.

Spicy Oat

Ingredients:

Oats (1/2 cup)

Brown rice (1/2 cup)

Dried oregano (1/4 cup)

Dried comfrey (1/4 cup)

Calendula (1/2 cup)

Myrrh (1/4 cup)

Anise seed (1/8 cup)

Clay (1 1/2 cups)

Lavender essential oil (1 drop)

Tea tree essential oil (1 drop)

Directions

Grind all ingredients except oils until powdery.

Add oils and then stir well.

Store in a jar.

To use: combine 1-2 teaspoon scrub and add a small amount of water.

Oatmeal Sunset Glow

The honey included in this scrub is a natural humectant. It absorbs moisture and keeps it under your skin —just where it ought to be. The apple cider vinegar restores your skin's natural acidity. Vinegar is ideal for both dry and oily complexions as it will keep it softy and fresh.

Ingredients

Oatmeal (8 tablespoons)

Apple cider Vinegar (1 tablespoon)

Dark organic Honey (1 tablespoon)

Finely ground Almonds (2 teaspoon)

Direction:

Put honey in a metal bowl or small glass then warm it in microwave till it becomes runny.

Mix all ingredients until you have a smooth paste

Seedy Oatmeal Body Scrub

Ingredients

Coarse rolled oats (1 handful)

Brown lentils (1 handful)

Jojoba oil (1/2 teaspoon)

Carrot oil (1/2 teaspoon)

Water

Directions

Blend the lentils in a blender until it is a coarse powder.

Add the rolled oats and blend to make powder. Add the oils and then process again.

Add water a teaspoon at a time until mixture becomes a thick paste.

Spoon into a container.

Oatmeal & Brown Sugar
A quick and gentle facial scrub

Ingredients

Brown sugar (2 teaspoon)

Fine colloidal oatmeal (2 tablespoon)

Citrus blend floral water (1 teaspoon)

Aloe moist (2 tablespoon)

Directions

1. Combine ingredients in a bowl until a smooth pasties achieved.

Oatmeal And More
The rich ingredients below is a peek of what to expect —it soothes, exfoliates, cleanse, moisturizes and more!

Ingredients:

Medium Cucumber (1/4 peeled)

Plain unflavored Yogurt (2 tablespoons)

Oatmeal (2 tablespoons)

Jojoba oil   (1 teaspoon)

Sweet Almond oil (1 teaspoon)

Direction:

Slice cucumber and whizz in food processor till it's liquefied.

Add remaining ingredients and mix to make a smooth paste.

Oats & Coffee

<u>Ingredients</u>

Rolled oats, chopped (1/3 cup)

Coffee grounds (2 teaspoon)

Raw honey (2 teaspoon)

Coconut oil (2 tablespoon)

<u>Directions:</u>

Combine all the ingredients in a bowl, mixing well.

Almonds, Avocado & Oatmeal

Use this avocado based scrub and see how smooth, soft, hydrated and nourished your skin will feel.

Ingredients:

Oatmeal (1 cup)

Coarsely ground Almonds (1 tablespoon)

Peeled ripe Avocado (1)

Direction:

Mix the grounded almonds and oatmeal. Next, mash the peeled avocado to a pulp.

Dip avocado pulp in the almond, oatmeal mix.

Rub and massage on your face very gently, then rinse off.

Coconut Oatmeal

Ingredients

Organic coconut oil (1/2 cup)

Oatmeal (1 1/2 cup)

Brown sugar (1 teaspoon)

Vanilla extract (1 teaspoon)

Honey (1 teaspoon)

Directions

In a food processor, ground oatmeal and place in a bowl.

Add brown sugar to finely ground oatmeal and then mix.

Pour vanilla, coconut oil and honey to the oatmeal and then mix until thoroughly combined.

Store in an airtight container.

Cheesy& Juicy Oatmeal

Cream cheese contains lactic acid that tones and cleanses the skin

Ingredients:

Oatmeal (2 tablespoons)

Cream cheese (1 tablespoon)

Fresh Lemon juice (1 teaspoon)

Direction:

Mix all ingredients until it forms a creamy paste.

Oatmeal &Peels

A rejuvenating scrub for those who want to smell fresh all day long

Ingredients:

Dried Orange peels (1 cup)

Oatmeal (1 cup)

Finely ground Almonds (2 tablespoon)

Sweet Orange essential oil (1 teaspoon)

Direction:

Put ingredients in a food processor and mix thoroughly. Take a little of this mix in your hand, add some warm water and make a paste. Rub and massage onto your skin.

Cornstarch, Oatmeal And More

A soothing and relaxing body scrub

Ingredients:

Almonds (1/4 cup)

Oatmeal (4 tablespoons)

Cornstarch (1 tablespoon)

Lavender essential oil (2 teaspoons)

Crushed dried Chamomile flowers (1 tablespoon)

Directions:

Place all ingredients in a food processor.

Blend and mash them well.

Take half a tablespoon of this mix in your hand. Add water to make a paste.

Milky Oatmeal

Ingredients

Whole milk (1 tablespoon)

Extra virgin olive oil (1 tablespoon)

Honey (1 tablespoon)

Oatmeal (2 tablespoon)

Directions

Combine ingredients in a bowl.

Leave for 5 to 10 minutes and then use.

Cucumber Oatmeal

Ingredients

1 cucumber (2 tablespoon cucumber paste)

Rosehip oil (1 teaspoon)

Argan oil (1 teaspoon)

Oatmeal (2 tablespoon)

Milk (1 tablespoon)

Directions

Blend cucumber in the blender to make a paste.

Add 2 tablespoon of the blended cucumber with the rest of the ingredients, mixing well.

Leave for about 5 minutes until oatmeal gets soft.

Use and discard leftover.

Cranberries, Coconut Super Oatmeal

Cranberries have everything your skin needs. Their inclusion in this recipe will help to exfoliate and clean your pores.

The coconut oil is not as greasy as other moisturizers. It is also very effective.

Ingredients

Cranberries (1/2 cup)

Oatmeal (4 tablespoons)

Coconut oil (2 tablespoons)

Sweet Almond oil (1 tablespoon)

Extra virgin Olive oil (1 tablespoon)

Brown Sugar (2 tablespoons)

Directions

Put ingredients in a food processor and mash and blend well.

The End

www.ingramcontent.com/pod-product-compliance
Lightning Source LLC
Chambersburg PA
CBHW020539290526
45786CB00002B/960